# Basic Ways to Get Over Anxiety, Depression, Anger.

By


ADEWUMI ADEDOYIN

# CONTENTS

# INTRODUCTION

Take heart if you've ever suffered from depression. Mindfulness, a simple but effective technique for paying attention to your most challenging emotions and life situations, can help you finally escape the cycle of persistent sadness. Four uniquely trained professionals explain why our customary attempts to "think" our way out of a poor mood or just "snap out of it" send us further into the downward spiral in The Basic Way through Depression. They teach how to avoid the mental patterns that lead to despair, such as rumination and self-blame, using profound lessons derived from both Eastern contemplative traditions and cognitive therapy, so you may confront life's obstacles with more resilience.

# WHAT IS DEPRESSION?

Depression is a mental health condition affecting millions of people worldwide. It is characterized by persistent feelings of sadness, hopelessness, and emptiness, as well as a loss of interest in once-enjoyable activities. Depression can be debilitating and impact every aspect of a person's life, from their relationships and work to their physical health.

There are many different types of depression, including major depressive disorder, persistent depressive disorder, and seasonal affective disorder. Each type of depression has its own unique set of symptoms and causes and may require different types of treatment.

Depression can be caused by a variety of factors, including genetic predisposition, environmental factors, and life events such as trauma or loss. Some of the most common symptoms of depression include feelings of sadness, hopelessness, and worthlessness, as well as fatigue, difficulty concentrating, and changes in appetite and sleep patterns.

Treatment for depression typically involves a combination of therapy and medication, although the exact course of treatment will depend on the individual's specific symptoms and needs. Therapies such as cognitive-behavioral therapy (CBT) and interpersonal therapy (IPT) can be effective in helping people manage their symptoms and develop coping skills, while medications such as selective serotonin reuptake inhibitors (SSRIs) can help regulate mood.

People with depression need to seek treatment as soon as possible, as the longer the condition goes untreated, the more severe the symptoms can become. Additionally, untreated depression can lead to other health problems, such as substance abuse, physical health issues, and even suicide.

If you or someone you know is struggling with depression, it is important to reach out for help. There are many resources available, including therapists, support groups, and crisis hotlines, that can provide guidance and support. With the right treatment and support, it is possible to manage depression and live a fulfilling life.

# WHY DEPRESSION IS THIS A PROBLEM?

Depression is a problem because it can significantly impact a person's quality of life and functioning in several ways. Some of the reasons why depression is a problem include:

- Negative impact on mental health: Depression can lead to persistent feelings of sadness, hopelessness, and worthlessness, as well as a loss of interest in once enjoyable activities. This can make it difficult for individuals to experience positive emotions or find pleasure in their lives.

- Impairment in daily functioning: Depression can make it difficult for individuals to perform everyday tasks such as getting out of bed, going to work or school, and maintaining social relationships. This can lead to problems in various areas of life, such as work, school, and personal relationships.

- Physical health problems: Depression can increase the risk of developing a variety of physical health problems, including heart disease, diabetes, and chronic pain. This can further impact a person's quality of life and ability to function.

- Risk of suicide: Depression is a significant risk factor for suicide, which is a leading cause of death globally. Individuals with depression may experience suicidal thoughts or behaviors, and they must receive appropriate treatment and support.

- Financial burden: Depression can lead to increased healthcare costs, as well as a loss of income due to reduced work productivity or unemployment. This can create a financial burden for individuals and their families.

Overall, depression is a problem because it can have a profound impact on an individual's mental and physical health, as well as their ability to function and participate fully in life. Individuals with depression need to seek treatment to manage their symptoms and improve their quality of life.

# WHAT DEPRESSION DOES TO THE BRAIN?

Depression can have a significant impact on the brain, and studies have shown that people with depression often have differences in brain structure and function compared to those without the condition.

**Here are some of the ways that depression can affect the brain:**

- **Alterations in brain structure:** Research has found that people with depression often have smaller volumes in certain areas of the brain, such as the hippocampus and prefrontal cortex. These brain regions are involved in regulating mood, memory, and other important functions.

- **Imbalances in neurotransmitters:** Neurotransmitters are chemicals in the brain that help to regulate mood and other functions. In depression, there is often an imbalance of certain neurotransmitters, such as serotonin and norepinephrine, which can contribute to symptoms of the condition.

- **Abnormalities in brain activity:** Brain imaging studies have shown that people with depression often have differences in the way their brains function compared to those without the condition. For example, there may be decreased activity in the prefrontal cortex, which is involved in regulating emotions and decision-making.

- **Impaired neuroplasticity:** Neuroplasticity refers to the brain's ability to change and adapt in response to new experiences. In depression, there may be impairments in neuroplasticity, which can make it more difficult for individuals to recover from the condition.

- **Increased inflammation:** There is growing evidence to suggest that depression is associated with increased inflammation in the brain and body. Chronic inflammation can damage brain cells and contribute to the development and progression of depression.

- **Neuroendocrine dysregulation:** Depression can also affect the function of the hypothalamic-pituitary-adrenal (HPA) axis, which is a key system involved in regulating the body's response to stress. In some people with depression, there may be abnormalities in HPA axis function, which can contribute to symptoms of the condition.

- **Impaired cognitive function**: Depression can also impact cognitive function, including memory, attention, and decision-making. These impairments may be related to changes in brain structure and function, as well as imbalances in neurotransmitters.

Overall, depression is a complex condition that can have wide-ranging effects on the brain. Understanding these effects is important for developing effective treatments and interventions for the condition, as well as for helping individuals with depression to manage their symptoms and improve their overall health and well-being

## WHICH DEPRESSION MEDICATION IS BEST?

There is no one-size-fits-all answer to which depression medication is the best, as different medications may work better for different individuals based on their specific symptoms, medical history, and other factors. Additionally, the effectiveness of a medication can vary depending on the severity of the depression and the individual's response to the medication.

That being said, several classes of medications are commonly used to treat depression, including:

- **Selective serotonin reuptake inhibitors (SSRIs):** SSRIs are often considered a first-line treatment for depression. These medications work by increasing the levels of the neurotransmitter serotonin in the brain, which can help to regulate mood. Examples of SSRIs include fluoxetine (Prozac), sertraline (Zoloft), and escitalopram (Lexapro).

- **Serotonin-norepinephrine reuptake inhibitors (SNRIs):** SNRIs work by increasing levels of both serotonin and norepinephrine, another neurotransmitter that is involved in mood regulation. Examples of SNRIs include duloxetine (Cymbalta) and venlafaxine (Effexor).

- **Tricyclic antidepressants (TCAs):** TCAs are an older class of antidepressants that work by increasing the levels of various neurotransmitters, including serotonin and norepinephrine. These medications can be effective, but they also have a higher risk of side effects compared to newer antidepressants. Examples of TCAs include amitriptyline (Elavil) and nortriptyline (Pamelor).

- **Monoamine oxidase inhibitors (MAOIs):** MAOIs are another older class of antidepressants that work by increasing levels of neurotransmitters in the brain. These medications can be effective, but they also have a higher risk of potentially dangerous interactions with certain foods and medications. Examples of MAOIs include phenelzine (Nardil) and tranylcypromine (Parnate).

In addition to these medications, other types of medications can be used to treat depression, such as atypical antipsychotics and mood stabilizers. Ultimately, the best medication for depression will depend on the individual's specific symptoms and medical history and should be determined in consultation with a qualified healthcare professional.

# NATURAL WAYS TO END DEPRESSION?

While medication and therapy are often effective treatments for depression, several natural ways may help alleviate symptoms or improve mood. Here are some natural approaches that may be helpful:

- **Regular exercise:** Exercise is an effective way to improve mood and reduce symptoms of depression. Even moderate exercise, such as walking or cycling, can have a positive impact. Exercise helps to release endorphins, which are natural feel-good chemicals in the brain.

- **Healthy diet:** Eating a healthy, balanced diet can also help to improve mood and reduce symptoms of depression. Focus on eating whole foods such as fruits, vegetables, lean proteins, and whole grains. Foods rich in omega-3 fatty acids, such as salmon and walnuts, may also be helpful.

- Mindfulness meditation: Mindfulness meditation involves paying attention to the present moment in a non-judgmental way. It is an effective way to reduce symptoms of depression and anxiety. There are many free resources available online to help you learn how to meditate.

- **Get enough sleep:** Getting enough sleep is essential for good mental health. Aim for 7-9 hours of sleep per night, and establish a regular sleep routine by going to bed and waking up at the same time each day.

- **Social support:** Spending time with friends and family and participating in social activities can be an effective way to improve mood and reduce symptoms of depression. Joining a support group or engaging in online forums can also provide a sense of community and support.

- **Yoga**: Practicing yoga can help to improve mood, reduce stress, and promote relaxation.

- **Acupuncture:** Acupuncture is a traditional Chinese medicine practice that involves inserting thin needles into specific points on the body to relieve pain and promote healing. Some research suggests that acupuncture may also help manage depression symptoms.

- **Massage therapy:** Massage therapy can help to reduce muscle tension, promote relaxation, and improve mood.

- **Aromatherapy:** Essential oils, such as lavender and peppermint, can be used in aromatherapy to promote relaxation and reduce stress.

- **Art therapy:** Engaging in art therapy, such as painting, drawing, or coloring, can be a helpful way to express emotions and reduce stress.

- **Music therapy:** Listening to music or playing an instrument can help to improve mood and reduce stress.

- **Dancing:** Dancing can be a fun and effective way to improve mood and reduce stress.

- **Spending time in nature:** Spending time in nature, such as going for a hike or spending time at the beach, can help to reduce stress and improve mood.

- **Pet therapy:** Spending time with animals, such as dogs or cats, can help to reduce stress and promote relaxation.

- **Herbal remedies:** Certain herbal remedies, such as St. John's wort and valerian root, may help manage depression symptoms. However, it is important to talk to a healthcare provider before using any herbal remedies, as they can interact with medications and cause side effects.

- **Gratitude journaling:** Writing down things you are grateful for each day can help to promote positive thinking and improve mood.

- **Cognitive-behavioral therapy:** Cognitive-behavioral therapy is a form of talk therapy that can help to change negative thinking patterns and improve mood.

- **Support groups:** Joining a support group, either in-person or online, can be a helpful way to connect with others who are experiencing similar challenges and receive emotional support.

- **Volunteer work:** Volunteering can help to improve mood and promote a sense of purpose and fulfillment.

- **Laughter therapy:** Laughter therapy involves engaging in activities that promote laughter, such as watching a funny movie or attending a comedy show. Laughter has been shown to have numerous physical and mental health benefits.

- **Tai chi:** Tai chi is a Chinese martial art that involves slow, gentle movements and deep breathing. It can help to promote relaxation and reduce stress.

- **Mind-body practices:** Mind-body practices, such as qigong and mindfulness-based stress reduction, can help to promote relaxation and reduce stress.

- **Writing:** Writing in a journal or writing creatively can be a helpful way to express emotions and reduce stress.

- **Social support:** Spending time with loved ones and connecting with others can help to reduce feelings of loneliness and improve mood.

- **Massage chairs:** Using a massage chair can help to reduce muscle tension, promote relaxation, and improve mood.

- **Float therapy:** Float therapy involves floating in a sensory deprivation tank filled with Epsom salt water, which can help to promote relaxation and reduce stress.

- **Light therapy:** Light therapy involves sitting in front of a special light box that emits bright light, which can help to regulate mood and reduce symptoms of depression.

- **Tapping therapy:** Tapping therapy, also known as Emotional Freedom Technique (EFT), involves tapping on specific points on the body while repeating positive affirmations. It can help to reduce stress and promote relaxation.

- **Herbal tea:** Drinking herbal tea, such as chamomile or lavender tea, can help to promote relaxation and reduce stress.

- **Spending time with children:** Spending time with children, such as playing games or doing

It is important to note that while these natural approaches can be helpful, they may not be sufficient for everyone with depression. If you are experiencing symptoms of depression, it is important to seek the advice of a qualified healthcare professional to determine the best course of treatment for you.

# HOW DOES DEPRESSION FEEL?

Depression is a complex condition that can manifest differently in different people. However, there are some common feelings and experiences that are often associated with depression. Here are some of the ways that depression may feel:

- **Persistent sadness:** People with depression may feel sad, empty, or hopeless for extended periods. This sadness may be intense and difficult to shake, and may not be related to any particular event or situation.

- **Lack of interest or pleasure:** People with depression may lose interest in activities they once enjoyed. They may feel like nothing is enjoyable or fulfilling anymore and may struggle to find pleasure in life.

- **Fatigue and low energy:** Depression can cause physical symptoms, such as fatigue and low energy. People with depression may feel like they don't have the energy to do even simple tasks and may feel exhausted even after getting enough sleep.

- **Negative thinking:** Depression can cause negative thinking patterns, such as self-criticism, self-blame, and feelings of worthlessness. People with depression may have difficulty seeing any positive aspects of their life and may feel like everything is going wrong.

- **Changes in appetite and sleep:** Depression can cause changes in appetite and sleep patterns. Some people may experience decreased appetite and weight loss, while others may experience increased appetite and weight gain. Similarly, some people may struggle to fall asleep or stay asleep, while others may sleep excessively.

- **Physical symptoms:** Depression can cause physical symptoms such as headaches, muscle pain, and digestive problems. These symptoms may not be related to any other underlying medical condition.

- **Feelings of worthlessness or guilt:** People with depression may feel like they are a burden on others, or that they are worthless. They may also feel guilty about things that are not their fault.

- **Difficulty concentrating or making decisions:** Depression can make it difficult to focus, concentrate, or make decisions. Even simple tasks may feel overwhelming, and it may be difficult to complete work or school assignments.

- **Suicidal thoughts or behaviors:** In some cases, depression can lead to suicidal thoughts or behaviors. People with depression may feel like life is not worth living or may feel like they are a burden on others. If you or someone you know is experiencing thoughts of suicide, it is important to seek immediate medical attention.

- **Irritability and restlessness:** Depression can also cause irritability and restlessness. People with depression may feel easily agitated or annoyed and may have a low tolerance for frustration.

- **Withdrawal from social activities:** People with depression may also withdraw from social activities, isolating themselves from friends and family. They may feel like they don't have the energy or motivation to engage with others, or may feel like others won't understand what they are going through.

- **Physical symptoms:** In addition to fatigue and changes in appetite and sleep, depression can cause a range of physical symptoms such as aches and pains, digestive problems, and headaches. These symptoms may not be related to any other underlying medical condition.

It is important to note that depression can manifest differently in different people, and not everyone with depression will experience all of these symptoms. If you or someone you know is experiencing symptoms of depression, it is important to seek the advice of a qualified healthcare professional to determine the best course of treatment.

It is also important to remember that depression is a treatable condition, and there are many effective treatments available. If you or someone you know is experiencing symptoms of depression, it is important to seek the advice of a qualified healthcare professional to determine the best course of treatment. With the right treatment and support, it is possible to manage depression and improve quality of life.

# HOW DOES DEPRESSION AFFECT STUDENTS?

Depression can have a significant impact on students, both academically and personally. Here are some of the ways that depression can affect students:

- **Academic performance:** Depression can make it difficult to concentrate, focus, and retain information. As a result, students with depression may struggle academically and may experience a decline in grades or academic performance.

- **Attendance:** Students with depression may be more likely to miss classes or skip school altogether. This can impact their academic performance and may make it difficult to keep up with coursework.

- **Social interactions:** Depression can make it difficult to engage with others and form social connections. Students with depression may withdraw from social activities and may struggle to make friends or maintain relationships with peers.

- **Self-care:** Depression can make it difficult to take care of oneself, including personal hygiene, exercise, and nutrition. Students with depression may neglect these aspects of their health, which can impact their overall well-being and academic performance.

- **Substance abuse:** Students with depression may be more likely to engage in substance abuse as a way of coping with their symptoms. This can lead to further problems, including addiction and academic or personal problems.

- **Increased stress:** Depression can make students more vulnerable to stress and anxiety. They may struggle to cope with everyday stressors, such as schoolwork, relationships, and family issues.

- **Decreased motivation:** Depression can make it difficult to feel motivated or engaged with schoolwork. Students with depression may feel like they have lost interest in their studies or may struggle to find the energy to complete assignments or projects.

- **Risk of suicide:** In some cases, depression can lead to suicidal thoughts or behaviors. Students with depression may feel like life is not worth living or may feel like they are a burden on others. If you or someone you know is experiencing thoughts of suicide, it is important to seek immediate medical attention.

Students with depression need to seek help and support from mental health professionals, as well as from family and friends. Treatment for depression may include talk therapy, medication, or a combination of both. In addition, lifestyle changes such as exercise, healthy eating, and stress management can also be effective in managing depression symptoms. With the right treatment and support, students with depression can learn to manage their symptoms and improve their overall well-being.

# WILL DEPRESSION EVER GO AWAY?

Depression is a treatable condition, and with the right treatment and support, many people can recover and manage their symptoms effectively. However, the duration and severity of depression can vary from person to person, and for some individuals, it may be a chronic condition that requires ongoing management.

It is important to seek professional help if you are experiencing symptoms of depression, as treatment can help you manage your symptoms and improve your quality of life. Treatment options may include therapy, medication, or a combination of both. Lifestyle changes, such as regular exercise, healthy eating, and stress reduction techniques, can also help manage symptoms of depression.

While depression may never fully go away for some individuals, with proper treatment and management, it is possible to lead a fulfilling life and reduce the impact that depression has on day-to-day activities. It is important to continue seeking support from a mental health professional and to develop coping mechanisms to manage depression symptoms.

It is also worth noting that depression can sometimes recur, even after successful treatment. In some cases, individuals may experience multiple episodes of depression throughout their lifetime. However, having experienced depression in the past does not necessarily mean that it will happen again. With proper treatment and management, individuals can reduce the risk of future depressive episodes.

It is important to take steps to maintain your mental health and well-being, even after recovering from depression. This may include continuing with therapy, taking medications as prescribed, making lifestyle changes, and seeking support from loved ones. Engaging in regular self-care activities, such as exercise, meditation, or hobbies, can also be beneficial in promoting mental wellness and reducing the risk of depression recurrence.

In summary, depression is a treatable condition, and with the right treatment and support, it is possible to recover and manage symptoms effectively. While depression may not necessarily fully go away for some individuals, ongoing management and self-care can reduce the impact that depression has on daily life and help individuals lead fulfilling lives.